HOW TO BE HAPPY

TRUE HAPPINESS is Made of 3 Pillars

*How to LIVE a Life of LOVE and be
HAPPY*

Simple and Easy Habits
Gain the WISDOM and KNOWLEDGE you Need

Dena S Moore

LIVE with gratitude
LOVE with a merciful heart
Be HAPPY for today

xoxoxo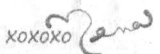

Thanks to God for blessing me with the Wisdom to pass along all that I have lived, loved and learned along my own happiness route. May your journey be a light in your life, and you experience and absorb all the wisdom you need along the way.

Dena Moore
Visit website at www.LiveLoveHappy.com
www.DenaSMoore.com

Printed in the United States of America

First Printing: May 2019
Live Love Happy

ISBN-9781080039821

ASIN: B07V6T8CL1

CONTENTS

TODAY IS AN EXCEPTIONAL DAY FOR BOTH OF US

Congratulations on taking the journey!

Let's get started! Stop what you are doing.

Smile   – hold for 2 seconds.

You are doing great, even if you did not make it the full 2 seconds. Believe it or not, getting started is truly the hardest part, even if it is relatively simple.

Are you ready for the best news ever? Being happy, getting happy, staying happy is not random, it is not by chance. You have control and can decide to take control. Even if you slip along the way it is easy to gain control, either a little bit at a time or all at once. This is the best news ever!

Now that I have your attention you may be ready to disagree with me and this is no surprise. Why? Because most people can argue that they were happy at other times in their life without trying. And you would be right. At those times, you were embracing something wonderful or in a different place, naturally doing and participating in activities that made you happy.

I used to think I was naturally happy; however, I am not, I just happened to naturally know the 3 pillars of happiness and actions to get, keep and stay happy.

Over the last 40 years of interacting, watching and listening to students, stay-at-home moms, college students, professionals, retirees, the poor, and the rich in everyday situations has allowed me to witness the universal, somewhat mysterious ways Happiness comes and goes. The elusiveness of Happiness appears to be a mystery; however, it isn't really. What if I told you there could be no more grasping for happiness or trying to hang onto happiness, that you could give it to yourself whenever you want happiness.

It is now my time to share with you how to create or expand your own Happy.

Smile —hold for 3 second then we will start your journey to a happier you. Seriously, stop and SMILE ☺.

Fair warning, on this journey, you will overwhelm yourself if you try to do all three of the pillars in the first days or weeks. I've grouped items together for a couple of different reasons. The initial groupings can be done by yourself, while the groupings later in the book involve more people or tasks that take a bit more effort. The most wonderful aspect of this book is that you can jump around as the situation best fits you and your life. <smile> You have control, isn't life great! If it isn't great now, keep working at it, practicing, taking on a new task or two every few days and you will soon increase your happiness creating a better, happy you.

Does it feel like Happiness is just out of reach; either just in front of you, behind you or sitting only in your friends' driveway. In all honesty, it is surrounding you and is yours for the taking. But you do have to work at it and take what is yours for the asking. Give yourself permission to be happy and be the happy for others. Believe me.... they need it and will appreciate it though it may take a while for them to figure it out.

We will start out with a few simple exercises before the main material.

Keep in touch through our Facebook group, website and emails to find out more about how to develop, grow, rekindle, find or simply learn more about happiness and how it can be yours all the days you want.
- www.LiveLoveHappy.com
- Facebook Group – Love Love Happy Life

MORE THAN YOU

Be the Inspiration - Motivation to Someone's Journey to Happiness

Welcome to your jump start to a happier life! Before we begin the journey, your route to happiness, always be on the lookout for opportunities to be the inspiration for someone else's happiness.

It has been proven time and time again that removing the focus from yourself will not only improve another persons' circumstance, in some if not all instances, your own life will benefit. Even though you may feel like there is nothing you have to give someone; a smile, kind word, or simply listening can often work wonders. Remember, do not judge a person or circumstance you may encounter. We often wear masks and the happiest person may be just the person that needs compassion, empathy or a smile the most.

Actions you can take immediately:
- When you are out, raise your head up and look around, notice your surroundings and the people
- You don't even have to look directly at someone, simply smile and nod your head as if you were acknowledging someone
- Don't be surprised when someone smiles back

CONGRATULATIONS ON STARTING YOUR JOURNEY

Your Route to Happiness

The smallest of changes consistently can lead to enormous benefits to your life. As you move through this book; the lessons, tasks, stories, and words of advice will take you far:

> *"Life is all about second, third and fourth chances; take as many*
> *Do-overs as needed."*

A hard part of understanding being happy is that you are responsible for your own happiness and only you can truly make your life a long one filled with happiness.

USE YOUR 5 SENSES

Simple Acts of Kindness

At times, one of the most difficult things to do when you aren't happy is being nice to someone else or doing something nice for someone else.

What do I mean by this?

Not some grand gesture, instead try a very small act that takes little or no effort.

Use your five senses to be aware and mindful allowing you to focus on the present and not the past or future which can weigh you down or cause undue stress. Take 5-10 minutes to live in the moment and bring awareness to the here and now. Watch the sunrise in the morning, hear the laughter around you, smell the air, taste the food or touch the side of your face as you smile.

Let your five senses help you become more aware of your surroundings and possibly find the opportunity to spread a bit of happiness to someone else.

SEE
As you are taking a walk in your neighborhood and enjoying your surroundings, you may hear the sweet chirping of birds calling out to one another. Listen for the buzzing of the bees as they fly from flower to flower gathering pollen to make delicious, sweet, gooey honey. Pay special attention to anyone else enjoying the outdoors and look up and smile at them. That simple smile may be the highlight of their day. When we reach out and touch or smell a flower, it may be enough of an action that someone else notices and may begin a conversation or a simple smile in each other's direction. If you normally keep your head down, try your best to lift it up and watch for the opportunity to give a smile away.

HEAR
As you listen to the click or shuffling of shoes going down the hallways, the buzzing of vibrating cell phones from co-workers passing by, conference calls and

the rushing sounds of going in and out of cubicles, try to catch someone's eye to give a quick nod and smile their way. In this very stressful environment, that simple smile may be the highlight of their day. If possible, reach out and shake someone's hand, thanking them for a job well done or let them know they are appreciated. If you normally keep your head down, try your best to lift it up and watch for the opportunity to give a smile away.

SMELL

Smells that will send your senses into wondrous delights; delicate aroma of oranges, sweet and tart cherries, that deep earthy rich smell as you bring tomatoes to your face, now look up and catch someone's eye to give a quick nod and smile their way. Whether you are at the local grocery, busy Walmart or the Farmer's Market, that simple smile may be the highlight of their day. Look around, raise your head, catch someone's eye and give a smile away.

TASTE

If there is a tasting booth at the grocery, local fair or farmer's market, simply thanking the person and finding a way to compliment them will often be the best thing they will hear all day. Walk up with a smile on your face, look around their items with interest. Try your best to smile and ask a question about something they are making or selling. Most people love to talk about what they have an interest in or like to do. This is the perfect opportunity to give a smile away.

TOUCH

A touch of a hand, a hug or warm and caring pat is often all it takes to make someone's day. Now add a smile to go with any of those and you will more than double the impact.

PAY IT NOW

Easy, Hard, Simple or Big

Throughout the day you may be asked, 'How are you?', or you may be the one asking someone else. If you ask someone 'How are you?' - STOP! Now from this day forward, when you ask someone, STOP, truly STOP moving your feet and your voice and take the time to listen to their answer about their day, their happy, sad or trying moments. Take the time to listen, rejoice in their joy, empathize and give understanding to the not so fortunate moments. The time that you take, whether it is 30 seconds or 5 minutes, could be the greatest act of kindness they receive simply because you chose to listen to them.

Remember the movie and the 'Pay It Forward' movement? Can you imagine instead of thinking of ways to pay it forward, we learned to live in a 'Pay It Now' world of just being nice, even if it is just with a small smile.

No action is too small to help lift someone on their journey to happiness, even if they don't know they are on one yet, you have begun yours.

The list is long on all the possibilities that you can do in the smallest of ways, or the largest of grand gestures; hailing a taxi for a stranger, helping the elderly in or out a door, saying thank you with sincerity, commenting on a stranger's T-shirt, asking your co-worker how their family is doing, thanking the cashier for the friendly smile and wonderful service. That simple act may be the highlight of their day.

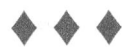

MY STORY

What's your Story?

I have ultimately been blessed much of my life, not because I was lucky, never had challenges or surrounded only by positive people or situations. In fact, if someone recounted some of the circumstances and events in my life, one might surmise that I was a bit unlucky, too often at the wrong place at the wrong time, simply a poor soul that needed a pat on the head.

So how in the world was it that I didn't feel that way, see myself that way or be over-whelmed by some of those circumstances? Keep reading and you will find out how you can create a better you, a happy way of life.

You will find out what the secrets are and how you can also take control to live a naturally happy life.

The habits you will learn will become second nature, however there will be days that you have to take control and do one or more of the 'happy' tasks on purpose.

There are still days that I must make the choice and take the route that puts me back on track to happiness by following my own advice. It is simple, however, not always easy. It could be that every day and sometimes every hour you must tell yourself to take on one of the Happiness Tasks. There have been occasions in the past that it was several times an hour I had to take on a task. Yes, this may involve talking to yourself on more than one occasion. Remember, it is never cool to yell at yourself, no one has time for that!

We all have stories, hurdles we overcame or need to overcome. How often does your day start then somewhere along the lines, Wham! you are hit with anxiety or anger that passes through you like unchecked rage due to someone's actions, words or circumstances. Surprises in our everyday lives that seem overwhelming, pull us down. Sometimes it isn't the daily grind, it is our lives as a whole, our situation whether it is family, environment, career or friends that pull us into a swirling drain of unhappiness.

HOW TO BE HAPPY

Sitting at the dining room table, reaching for the last piece of chicken, cake or bread, remembering the deep smell of warm brownies as I ate more than I should led me to be the fat girl, teased, called names and bullied for a time in my life. The laughs and giggles of two little blonde children, playing with dolls and paperclips, swimming, games of chase and mismatched socks, little darlings the highlight of my life, was a result of being a pregnant teen mom. Days in which I am sure there wasn't enough of my patience to go around. Living the white picket fence dream, the fairytale that was ripped away in a very ugly divorce. A beautiful new house, out in the country, beautiful yard and spectacular views that was also the home of a nest of deadly, poisonous brown recluse spider. The bites took me years to overcome, however I was so thankful and grateful that my kids were not bitten. On my own, kids grown, I bravely packed a backpack, left the country and went on an adventure. Let's just say I was totally unprepared and found myself kidnapped in a foreign country and I was extremely lucky in this horrific experience because I could buy my way to freedom, others, I am sure have not been as fortunate. In the land of the Free and Brave, I found myself betrayed by one of the most symbolic of companies in America, Disney, my co-workers and I fired in my fifties and replaced by cheap foreign labor that I had to train. Then there were the normal incidents in life; the multiple car accidents throughout the years, working through fears of heights (otherwise known as 'fear of falling'), battling claustrophobia and you know, normal family and friends' drama. Believe me, these are just a few hurdles that popped up for me. Everyone has stories, some not as dramatic as mine and others much, much worse. These may be minor to what you have experienced, or they may be more than you can comprehend.

I am going to share with you the secrets, actions and tasks that not only helped me overcome, but propelled me into a future filled with happiness. Because of these habits, the happiness habits, the tasks that you can also follow so that nothing can stand in your way, nothing can impact you very long because the happiness habits will help you succeed. My wish for you is that you turn any obstacle that comes your way, any setback, any negative event into just a minor hiccup that you do not even recognize it as it is happening to you.

Enough about me, let's continue down your new road, your journey to happiness and a happier, better life.

A side note on medical depression. There are some people that do have a chemical imbalance and I encourage anyone that feels that they may suffer from clinical depression or anxiety to see their doctor to be tested. Most of us do not have

9

a chemical imbalance and we don't need medication to achieve happiness or remove a depressing outlook, attitude or anxiety. However, it does take more effort, especially in the beginning to learn the skills, practice the tasks and become a naturally happy person. For those that need medication for chemical imbalances, sometimes the medication is not enough and the efforts to follow the 3 pillars of happiness are also necessary. So, if you find yourself taking prescribed medications for anxiety or depression, and still feel lacking in happiness, then keep reading, participate in the tasks, take the steps to complete your journey that may just result in a happier you.

EASY AND ONLY YOU

(Hope)

These next few chapters may seem to be the easiest because they only involve you.

This will also make them at times the hardest because they only involve you, so you must force yourself to reach deep down, even if you do not want to and carry out these next few tasks.

To some these tasks are small, while to others they may seem or feel like mountains.

As you read each task, know that there are many people traveling on this journey with you and could easily be the person in front, beside or behind you. Welcome to this journey, it will be fun, easy, simple, difficult, short and sometimes long. You are worth it and pretty soon you will know what true happiness really looks like.

AUTOPILOT

Just Say NO!

The story of missing time. Have there been days, hours, minutes that you missed out on because you zoned out and went into autopilot?

Have you ever gotten to work, racing to catch the elevator, sometimes catching it and other times, not so much.? Checking the time, you realize you may be late as you are juggling your car keys, almost dropping everything, including the piping hot coffee you just bought? Can you fully recall your commute to work, or is it a bit fuzzy? On tomorrow's commute, stay tuned, watch for the details and enjoy finding something you haven't seen before.

What if halfway through your day you could win $1000 if you could recall what your spouse, son, daughter or friend was wearing the last time you spent time with them? Tell me the last compliment you gave to one of your family, friends and spouse.

Have you ever noticed the dishwasher had run and you don't remember turning on? Or how many times have you turned around to go back home to check on a garage door not shut, coffee pot left on, security alarm not set before you had control through your phone.

Many things escape our attention because we simply don't tune in to our lives. I wonder how much time is lost to being on autopilot? You know, you have a choice to participate, to live in those moments.

Great joy can be found in the smallest details. Are you ready to learn how to control your autopilot?

Decide today to catch yourself during or before you zone out.

Write down 3 things that you can do when you catch yourself zoning out and not living in the moment.

Becoming aware when you are zoning out.

This is the first key and then following it with a behavior, task or thought.

Choose one of the examples below, or create one of your own each time you catch yourself:

- Smile that you caught yourself going into or coming out of an autopilot zone.
- Whistle out loud
- Turn up the radio and sing
- Talk to the person closest to you
- Snap your fingers
- Tap your toes
- Wink

In order to fully live each minute, hour and day, zoning out is not an option. First catch yourself, then ask yourself why you zoned-out. Often it is because of boredom, not wanting to listen or be a participant in an activity. Once you have caught yourself zoning-out, begun a behavior, thought or task each time you caught yourself and figured out the why you were zoned-out, you can break free and begin paying more attention to life around you.

Paying attention to the details or have an activity will stop the boredom zone-out. Actively participating, finding the good, interesting or fun will stop the 'I wish I wasn't here zone-out'. Life is not supposed to be lived on Auto-pilot, take control beginning today.

NOT AS SIMPLE AS IT SEEMS

Getting out of Bed

Are there some mornings, afternoons or evenings that you simply want to pull the covers over your head and not get out of bed? Is it a contest to see how many times you can hit the snooze button?

Believe it or not, this is often the easiest challenge to overcome. Why? Because this is on you, not anyone else. This is the start of your day, nothing has happened to impact your day, it is just you, your thoughts, your choice of sabotage or courage.

You are the only one accountable for the outcome.

If you find yourself in this predicament, decide three small tasks that you are going to do right away. For these tasks, sometimes it is best not to choose what you must get done, but three small things that are nice to do or are options for the day. It is often the things that you must do that are making you want to hide your head.

So how does this help?

Once you are up and accomplishing something, you will find that you rarely want to just jump back into the bed. These small successful tasks turn on your brain, create success and positive emotions.

Sample of small tasks:
- Text a friend good morning
- Check and clear out all junk email
- Clear up last night's dishes
- Play 5-10 minutes of your favorite game
- Post 'Good Morning' on your social media account
- Meditate for 5-10 minutes

- Send a friend a compliment via phone call, text, messenger or any other means

You make the choice every day to get up and get started. Most days you probably just do it automatically, however there are probably some days or a time in your life that you just don't want to. Everyone has these days, now you know what to do when you must take control on those days to get going. Choose your path to Happiness instead of pulling the covers up over your head.

Note: you will often find yourself talking to yourself about just getting up, not to stay in bed, put your feet on the floor and move. The first steps are the hardest, but it is the one thing that is totally up to you.

WHAT'S IN A SMILE?

More than Lips and Teeth

How about something easy and can be done anywhere?

What I am about to ask you to do is so easy you may not even feel it is necessary, however don't be fooled with its simplicity.

Not much is needed for this exercise; a mirror, any will do, even if it is just something reflecting your face. I have been known to use the reflective handle on my refrigerator, my reflection in a window, 1980s mirror sunglasses, no excuses if a real mirror is not handy.

Before you go out in the world you must practice all the faces of a Smile; from the small lip only smile to the middle smile that only shows a bit of your teeth, to the full-fledged smile in which a laugh may also be involved.

Once you have this down, go out in public anywhere, this especially works where you know absolutely no one.

Now, as you pass strangers, simply deploy one of your smiles. Sometimes nodding your head while smiling. Pull out your phone as if speaking to a friend and give the good hearty belly laugh and smile all the while looking around. You will see people respond, simply nod and give them one of your smaller smiles.

So, you may say or think, what does this do for me. Nothing!

Not in the immediate at least, but the effect you may have had on the person receiving your gift or the ripple effect on how it impacted their day or the people they meet in the course of their day.

Believe it or not, until it becomes natural for you to just smile and nod to people, you may feel exhausted. Now I know that some of you will think this is crazy, while others totally get the need for a cup of coffee or alone time after this adventure.

Trust me, this simple way of living; smiling at most people you pass by, even if they don't seem to see you will change not only their life, but yours over time.

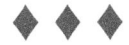

3 PILLARS THAT MAKE UP TRUE HAPPINESS

True Happiness =
Meaningful Life + Purpose + Pleasure

Feelings of Meaning = a Meaningful Life

Purpose = Your Why in Life

Pleasure = joy, gratitude, serenity, interest, hope, pride, amusement, inspiration, awe, satisfied, delight, gladness, glee, content, enjoyment, love and happy

Have you said to yourself or heard others say they want to be happy?

Have you often felt you were happy and then within seconds something came along and stole your happiness right out from under you?

There is a difference between 'True Happiness' and 'Being Happy'. Most people go after 'Being Happy' and don't understand that in order to acquire the everlasting happiness you must learn how to go after and obtain 'True Happiness'.

'Being Happy' comes from pleasure. Pleasure can be fleeting, constantly needs fed by one or more of the pleasure actions. You will exhaust yourself if you tried to keep yourself happy with pleasure.

Most people miss out on keeping their Happiness because they only have one element of Pleasure of the True Happiness formula. The one item that is random or constantly has to be worked on is Pleasure; that momentary, fleeting things that happen causing one of the pleasure feelings to appear. If True Happiness was only based on pleasure, life would feel like a roller coaster. WAIT, WAIT, WAIT!!!!

Save the roller coasters for the amusement park, take control of your happiness by learning the 3 pillars and how to control the pleasure, meaning, and purpose along with actions that will enable you to have, find and grow your 'True Happiness'

Most people have been taught that happiness is simply Pleasure which is why so many people in the world are in search of their happiness. Most people are waiting for something to happen to make them happy, waiting on someone else to do something to make them happy, mad because something happened that brought about another emotion and stole their happy, making them even more unhappy. Sound familiar?

Being happy engages many of your feelings and emotions and they play a vital role in maintaining your happiness.

The key to true, lasting happiness is to build a solid foundation with Pillar #1, A Meaningful Life and Pillar #2, Purpose and your Why and Pillar #3, Pleasure which is not as easy as it sounds because it covers things you have to work at and put forward effort.

In order to be and stay happy you must build and create Pillar #1, a Meaningful Life. The main emotion behind a Meaningful Life is Pride.

Pillar #2 is fulfilled by discovering your Purpose and Why. The main emotions behind Purpose and Why are inspiration, love and joy.

Pillar #3 is comprised of several parts and there are many emotions tied to pleasure; joy, gratitude, serenity, interest, hope, pride, amusement, inspiration, awe, satisfied, delight, gladness, glee, content, enjoyment, love and happy.

Throughout this book you will be taught how to create your own pleasure, a very important and key element that needs to be added on a consistent basis. The next two Pillars that are essential for your journey to Happiness is creating and understanding Feelings of Meaning and finally discovering, defining and always looking towards your purpose(s).

PILLAR #1: FEELINGS OF MEANING

(pride)
Meaningful Life

You are superb, thank you for getting this far on your journey. Not only am I proud of you, you should be very proud of yourself.

Now, what else can you tell me that would make me proud of you?

Were you especially nice to someone, help someone, thank someone? Did you take care of yourself today? Did you improve today putting away some negativity? Did you change the subject when someone began chatting about something negative? Did you smile today?

From the smallest to the largest effort, doing something and taking pride in it, or because of it will go a long way to reaching your happy. Don't brush off the little things, it is these things that can make you stand taller, puff your chest up a bit and make your day feel a bit lighter and brighter.

Many, many times we forget to pat someone on their back; including ourselves. In this busy, busy world sometimes you must be your own cheerleader.

The role you play in your family should also be a large part of creating a meaningful life for yourself. Remember, family can mean immediate family, friends that are close as family or even your city, state or country family. If you have never thought of having pride and growing your self-worth through your family, friends, associations, work, hobbies and interests, now would be a great time to start.

Now that you know that taking pride in something, whether it is small, medium or large, will take you fast to your happy, perhaps you will remember to tell someone you meet or know that you are proud of them. Don't assume that they know you appreciate them or what they are doing. You never know, this may bring awareness for them and cause them to thank or appreciate someone else, on and on bringing on a avalanche of happiness. How grand would that be?

Let's look into the key areas of our lives and put a meaningful life aspect to it, opening our eyes, minds and heart to the pride we can bring to each of these areas.

MEANINGFUL FAMILY AND HOME LIFE

Family and Home

Family

Let's start with family, which can be immediate, extended and even what I call family plus, those people that are friends and as dear as family. Those people in your life that are more than friends. Often referred to this as sisters from another mister or brothers from another mother.

It is easy to quickly dismiss how important your role is in your family and to your friends. Take a few minutes and make a list, even if it is only mentally, on what your role is to your family and friends. Below are some ideas and questions that will help you become aware of what it takes to create a meaningful life with family and friends.

If you have a spouse and children:
- Do you take care of things around your house, apartment, flat, condominium or yard?
- Do you help provide meals?
- Do you read, have conversations, or help with homework if you have children?
- Do you give hugs, smiles and words of encouragement?

If you have extended family:
- Do you call and check on your mom, dad, auntie, uncle, cousins, brothers, sisters?

- Do you send cards, notes or small gifts?
- Do you drop by for a visit?
- Do you run errands, take care of things?

Home:
- Do you help clean and provide a safe environment?
- Do you make your bed? (either in the morning or before you get in bed at night)
- Do you provide a clean environment for yourself and family?
- If you have pets, are they well cared for?

The questions above are just a few examples to help you realize that you are helping provide for others in your family or friends. All of these contribute to a meaningful life, bringing not only satisfaction into your life, it brings happiness, contentment and smiles into the lives of others.

One of the best ways to create a more meaningful life is to do MORE THAN your fair share when it comes to family and friends.

Ask yourself, 'Are you doing more than your fair share to support, improve and work towards the best family and friend's life you can have?'. Just think if everyone did more than their fair share how much nicer life would be for everyone.

Remember, this is just a starter list of things for you to think about. See Live-Love-Happy Blog for a longer list of ideas to help increase Home, Family and Friends meaningful life ways of living. A meaningful life may start out as a checklist but will soon become a way of life and put you well on your way to a Happier Life.

If you were one of the many people that read through the list and thought to yourself; uh oh, I don't do very many or any of the items listed, do not despair. The wonderful news is that this ingredient of creating Happiness can start at any time, it is never too late.

When you read this information on a Meaningful Life, it may seem like these ideas are really easy to incorporate or expand in your life, which they are if everyone would take some time to carry them out. However, perhaps they are too easy as there are many people who do not make the most of living a meaningful life when it comes to family and friends.

It may be time for you to increase your efforts in the things you do, however small when it comes to your family and friends. You may never realize how much impact a simple email, hand-written note, phone call to a near or distant family member or friend will make. Whether you choose to tidy up, write a love note or a simple smiley on a post-it note, start today to increase your value within your family and friends circle.

MEANINGFUL WORK LIFE

Work

Work – Deciding what you do and why it matters

You know, work is always a topic that has caused much controversy and dissatisfaction for many people.

There is a very simple explanation for this phenomenon. There are so many advertisements, articles and advice that you should only work in a job that you love or doing something you love to do.

What if I told you that was bad advice? Before you stop reading and try to dispute this statement, have a quick read, then try what I am asking you to try and keep an open mind. Let me explain about why it is bad advice. It sets you up for failure, either because you cannot find a job that pays you to play music, write, kayak, or text all day. You then become discontent, unhappy or always grumbling that you cannot find or make money doing the thing you love.

Do not forgo your dream, keep working at what you love. Work really hard at getting better at what you love. Take pride in your abilities, look for opportunities to expand your dream. If there is a chance to volunteer using your talent, by all means, jump at the volunteer opportunities. Do not give up on any possibility of obtaining your dream job, because it may be around the corner. Until that happens, do not fret, do not get depressed or complain that you do not have your dream job.

In the meantime, love what you are currently doing for work and smile while you are doing it. Look for every single benefit to your job.

The benefits may not be just for you getting paid, having the security of having a job, getting a few time off or even having health care. The position you currently hold with your employer may be helping someone's life be better, improving someone's situation, helping make money for your company so that you will be able to have and keep your job.

Think about this, if you acted happy to do your job, smiled while you were doing it, being grateful that you are helping yourself and others; do you think you will come across as a happier person?

At the end of every day, you should be able to pat yourself on the back for a job well done. Think about the good you did for someone by showing up and doing your best work.

Take pride in the fact that you showed up and gave your all that day, that week, that month.

If this isn't the job you think you want, then take the necessary steps to better yourself in order to make the change happen. However, in the meantime, be grateful, give it your all and love what you are doing for the here and now.

MEANINGFUL LIFE WITH FRIENDS

Friends

Friends:

Friendships come and go over your lifetime and some friendships last for a lifetime. The good news is that on any given day, if you want you can begin forming new friendships. For some, especially the group of people that do not have family, friends can become part of your family.

Building and working on friendships is crucial to creating and maintaining a meaningful life. As with family, your life becomes part of a building block Lego type system. You want your life to be independent, yet some nice dependencies on others and build relationships that have a dependency on you. This responsible act of making friends and maintaining friendships creates an interdependency amongst everyone.

A challenge that is often brought up is the challenge of being a loner or someone that just doesn't like to have close friendships. For this group of people even though it may seem challenging, it really isn't if you know the secrets to adapting friendships to your lifestyle. One way for you to remain a loner yet build the dependencies you need to build a meaningful life is to volunteer for a group within your community, or your hobbies or interests. This way even if you do not actually socialize with others, the group becomes dependent on your participation and you have created a responsibility to show up and do your part for the group.

You may have a challenge with how to make new friends because you have moved to a new place and you have left your friends behind. Always keep in touch with the friends you make along the way in life. In this day and age, it is so very easy to stay in touch with each other if you simply take the time. Planning a yearly weekend visit to your old stomping grounds or creating a group email to catch-up on everyone's life. One of the most fantastic ways to meet new friends is through real-life meet and greets, not just social media. Using social media, such as Meetup.com, to find groups is great because you don't just chat online, you actually meet out.

Friends:
- Do you call, text or email your friends on occasions in which you don't need anything?
- Do you know and remember friends on their birthdays; whether this is singing a birthday song, sending a birthday card or better yet going to see them in person?
- Do you set aside time each week or month to spend time with friends?
- Are you there for your friends when they are having a challenging time?

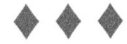

PILLAR #2: THE PURPOSE AND WHY

(Inspiration, love, joy)

Your Purpose

So, do you really want to be Happy? Seriously, do you enjoy being the person that people want to avoid, do you want to be the complainer of everything? Do you want to be the know-it-all? If you answer YES to these questions you may as well stop reading.

If you want to be happy, then let's chat about your purpose to getting, having, growing and experiencing your happiness.

There are so many benefits to being happy, so what is your purpose for experiencing, living and giving happiness?

For some, finding, knowing, developing your purpose will be quite easy, for others it may take some serious thinking and working through some of the steps to fully understand and embrace your purpose.

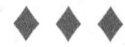

WHAT'S IMPORTANT CREATES PURPOSE

(Inspiration, love, joy)

Family, Friends, Acquaintances, Groups

The last chapters reviewed how a meaningful life plays an important part in being happy for life. This section though closely related to a meaningful life focuses on how your purpose affects your ability to have and sustain happiness in your life.

Whereas a meaningful life is about realizing your family, friends, acquaintances, groups, city, state and country, as examples, are one of the key factors in achieving true, lasting happiness. A meaningful life is learning how to be a quality part of a group, whether big or small that brings you pride.

Many people seem to have great difficulty finding their purpose in life, when it is quite easy. The biggest challenge or hurdle to get over is realizing you do not have to have just one big purpose in life. Start small by building on the meaningful things in your life. Having a purpose within a group is a much bigger commitment than just being a part of the group. Finding a purpose within a group is easy, just decide something to try that you think might inspire you, something you love or will find joy doing.

One of the easiest ways is to think about one of your personality traits:

- Are you outgoing? – Be the coordinator of activities to call, text or group chat others
- Are you organized and a planner? – Research and find possible activities the group will be interested in and then get with the outgoing person to let them communicate with the group

31

- Are you compassionate? Finding out other members in the group birthdays, anniversaries and special dates of members of the group and sending cards, emails, text messages or calls to wish them the best
- Are you artistic? Finding a way within your group to use your talent to help the group

It is truly up to you to make a commitment to be a bigger part of one or more groups you belong to and be the person that others can count on. You do not have to make this kind of commitment to every group you belong to and you can change your mind if you do not really care for the first, second or even third area you tried.

In this day and age, so many people think they do not want a commitment and so they are constantly running after being happy. A commitment that you enjoy creates a situation that people count on and builds on your purpose. This purpose gets better and better over time and will give you such a sense of pride that you stand a bit taller, your smiles get a bit bigger and others come to count on you to fill that bit of their lives within the group. This is truly your base for happiness.

A hurdle that you may have to overcome is if you choose the wrong area or thing to commit to along the way. This is so much easier that it seems, simply choose something else. Yes, it is truly that easy.

Being a part of a group or many groups gives you the opportunity to grow by meeting new people, having new experiences and even develop new skills or uncover skills you didn't know existed. The opportunity to develop a life with meaning and purpose is the foundation to true lifelong happiness.

Even if you have been a part of a group or many groups for a long time and only showed up or participated, there is always time to make a bigger commitment to develop a purpose within the group. Knowing and having your purpose is so often confused as a single thing, or individual want or desire.

Expand your thoughts beyond yourself, even if ultimately you find your purpose is to create something based solely upon your talents, being a part of a group could possibly lead to great opportunities, not to mention great friendships and fun times.

WHAT IF YOU COULD CHANGE SOMEONE'S LIFE?

(Inspiration, love, joy)

What's Important Creates Purpose

The emotional ties to living a life with purpose is inspiration, love and joy. To some people this will mean doing things that are inspirational to them, gives them joy or is something they love. If you want to live a bigger, deeper, happier life; do things that inspire others, brings love and joy to the lives and hearts of others.

Do you want to build your happiest life on a rock-solid foundation that cannot be shook no matter what comes your way? If so, make sure that you include in your life the things that create inspiration, exude love and compassion in others and joy that can be felt, seen and heard. Have you ever heard, "It's simple, just not always easy"?

Most people think they must plan or do something big to make an impact. The big things often start as a very small gesture that continually builds. So much time is spent thinking, researching and planning that nothing is ever began because it simply seems too hard or is put aside for another day. There is a saying 'Ready, Aim, Fire', what if we were all taught; 'Fire, Ready, Aim'. Using this concept, everyone would just do something then adjust along the way to improve the process.

Exactly how do you inspire someone else? There are so many different ways this can be done; however, the number one way is to live your life with purpose and share your stories and experiences with others. Another way is to take a true interest in people in your life and talk with them about what interests them. Simply taking a keen interest in another person's hobby or work will often inspire additional creativity, joy, pride and motivation in them to do better and be better.

Compliments are the truest way to spread joy to someone. Complimenting something they have created, accomplished or participated in will spark conversation, stories that will lead to reliving moments of joy and love. The building blocks of happiness are made stronger through reliving the joyous and lovely moments. As a person relives through the telling of the stories and tales, pride and purpose also strengthens which is the very foundation of happiness and their foundation is made stronger and stronger. Now that you know that repeating these stories works for others, start today making a list of all the stories you have to tell and share. Everyone loves a 'remember when' story.

There is a great deal of lives changed without the knowledge of the person who actually caused the change. You may be telling a story about one of your life adventures that inspires, motivates and causes change in another person's life at the time of the tale, or years' later down the road. A kind word or conversation may even be over heard that changes another's outlook and changes the course of their lives. Now that you know that these un-noticed positive actions can be the cornerstone in changing another persons' life, beware of your negative actions and words, because these can also cause unwanted, devastating changes to a stranger, dear friend or acquaintance.

Is there something that you are truly passionate and knowledgeable about and is positive? How often to you search out those like-minded people or groups? Do you take the opportunity to share your knowledge? What if you shared your knowledge through stories, demonstrations, one-on-one friendship get-togethers? When you do this, you will find that somewhere along this path that you will give someone a purpose, excite them beyond anything that has excited them before. In them you will see that this was just the inspiration, motivation, knowledge and excitement that they needed to add meaning and purpose to their lives. Through all of this not only is their foundation of happiness building and getting stronger, so is yours.

SELF – DREAM AND DREAM BIG

(Inspiration, love, joy)

Discovering what you want in life is simple, however, it is not the easiest of tasks. We may all 'want' quite a few things, some of them just a whimsy as they pass by our eyes, others we have been working towards for a short or long time. The task that you are about to embark on is more than a whimsy, an immediate desire or long list of items. What you are about to undertake will probably change your life forever because we are about to learn how to truly dream big, which is set to bring inspiration to your imagination, love and joy to your heart and head.

Before we begin to dream BIG about what we want in life; whether it is about spirituality, family, home, career, fun and adventure, we must clear our mind and let the noise of the day fall away. Let's start by practicing together as we begin to envision and dream about a place that we want to live sometime in the near or distant future.

Dream Exercise #1 – Home:
The Journey:

As we begin this journey of how to dream big, we will begin with a dream of where we may want to live in the future. Because we are reading, we will keep our eyes open, however when you are dreaming your big dream, after you know how, you may want to close your eyes. Now most people who dream small start with what kind of house/apartment/condo you are dreaming about, in order to have the biggest dream possible we won't start there. Instead, we will begin with the drive on the way to your new home; what kind of road are you driving on, is it a high speed highway, making your way through lively downtown traffic, a winding, mountain road with majestic trees covering the road, a scenic road with rolling hills passing by delicate grapevines, a sandy beach highway of tropical paradise? As you are driving to your new home, is the sun warming your heart, is the cool, brisk air causing you to zip or button up your jacket or is the air you breath forming miniature clouds to appear around your face. As we are making our way to your home, close your eyes and feel how fast, slow, cautious, reckless, you are traveling and the sights, sounds and smells that are passing by your eyes. This picturesque drive to your home is fundamental to the foundation of your inspiration and joy. Using all of your senses, what do you feel, hear, see and smell on this journey to your home.

Narrative:

As we practice using and growing our imagination for what our heart truly desires, you will begin to understand we are going starting with a big picture and taking it down to the smallest detail. By doing this you will uncover truths within yourself about what you really like, what experiences put a smile on your lips and joy in your heart. Instead of just thinking you want something, first go through the exercise of feeling what it is like to have it, own it, use it and mastering it. If you cannot take the time to embrace the item, task, or adventure, then surely it cannot be that important in your life.

What you will also find out about yourself by performing the exercise about the 'Journey to your Home' is aspects about the type of person you are and the life that excites you. For example, you may have envisioned a journey in the busy city, or the tranquility of the country, or perhaps even arriving to your home via a helicopter, boat or ship. The journey alone will tell you a lot about yourself. Keep going as we find out more about yourself.

The Ride:

Now that we are well along our way to your home, it is time to not only imagine the scenery you are passing by, but also the very vehicle that is taking you home. What kind of seat are you sitting in? What kind of noise is the engine making if there is even an engine? Reach out and touch what is in front of you, is it plush, shiny and hard, is there all kinds of gadgets? Are you going slow, fast, or super-fast? Are you walking, biking, riding, flying, floating to get there? Every detail is important as you detail out every color, texture and sound inside and outside on this journey. What clothes are you wearing? Is it hot, cold, summer, winter, dry, wet? Who, if anyone, is on this journey with you? Remember, this is your future self, do not limit yourself to your current situation. If you are not alone, are those with you friends, family, kids? Now try to define all the noises inside and outside of the vehicle.

Narrative:

As you can see, simply the ride to get to your dream home causes you to use so much of your imagination. As you begin to 'see', you may discard somethings that pop into your mind as a clear, vivid picture begins to form in your head and heart while seeing yourself traveling to get to your dream home. Is the ride exciting, leisurely, full of surprises, feel like an old pair of shoes you have had for ages, or new experiences around every corner?

The Entrance:

Time to pick up where we left off in your imagination as we approach the entrance to your dream home. Slow down and take in all the sights to see as we begin to approach the driveway or yard. For some of you there may be numerous flowers and fruit trees that have gorgeous smells as you pass by, for others there may be statues, pools or sophisticated gardens, while still other may be entering garage structures or land via boat or plane. Take the time to imagine every detail from the shape of every tree, stone and rock, decorative landscape or building structures on the property. Take note of the date, whether it is morning, mid-day or night, including whether it is sunny, cloudy or raining. How does the air smell, is it a windy or still day?

Narrative:

Each part of these imagination exercises brings out parts of your personality which drives your joy and love if you take the opportunity to imagine all details. You may find that you are experiencing a peace and calming about yourself or even be in amazement at some of the things that are so important to you that you did not realize before this journey.

The Outside of your Home:

Let's pick-up where we left off and get out of the vehicle that brought us to our dream home. Imagine you are barefoot, what is underneath your feet as you step out? Now that you know what the ground feels like, slowly raise your head and tell me what the first thing you see is? What is the first smell that hits your nostrils? Go through every detail of the exterior of your dream home, do not skip anything. How big or small is the doorway, what is it made of, is there a doorbell or windows? What kind of welcome mat is at the door if any? Can you count the windows, big, small, square, round, rectangle or no windows at all? Do not skip over any details, know the color or colors of the exterior. Do you hear or see birds chirping, butterflies and ladybugs flitting about, perhaps there is a boat, waterfall or wave whispering in the background?

Narrative:

At this point we haven't even made it into your home, this will come next. This simple journey using your imagination to truly discover your dream home, not only gives you imagery of the home you want in the future, it also takes you through the ideal road, vehicle and people you want to surround yourself with along this path of discovery. We spend so much time and energy before imagining the interior of your dream house for a couple different reasons. The first is to get your imagination jump-started towards bigger ideas and to walk you through the journey. It is always the journey that takes the longest, rushing to get to the end result will often leave you unhappy and miserable because you did not take the time and put your imagination to work to paint the picture, think through all the colors and details, for it is the journey that tells you the most about yourself. When using your imagination, it adds to your motivation and inspiration and should lead you to joy and love as you discovery truly who you are and what you really want in life, all which leads to happiness.

The Inside of your Home:

You have made a spectacular journey so far getting to your dream home, embracing the ride, arriving, envisioning the exterior. It is now time to open the door and go inside. Walk through each room, one at a time, imagining every wall, every knick knack, each piece of furniture, the flooring; whether it is soft or hard, patterned or plain and the feeling each room brings to your head and heart. Whether it is a grand home, a cozy cottage, a sailboat, apartment or tent out in the wilderness, imagine sight and smell. Imagine yourself reaching out and touching everything you imagine.

Narrative:

This journey should have tapped into every bit of your imagination and will have inspired you to look into the life you want to have that will bring joy and love to your heart. Looking beyond the physical things you imagined, this journey alone should have told you a great deal about yourself that maybe you have not yet come to realize. Was the journey fast and exciting or slow and relaxed? Was the trip by car, boat, airplane or something else, including perhaps hiking to your home? Even the exterior and interior of your home should have told you a great deal about who you really are.

This simple exercise can help you understand more about yourself and whether you are seeking out and participating in the activities, career and friendships that inspire you bringing you joy and love. These moments of 'Oh Yea! That's me!' will be built on throughout your life, no matter when you discover them.

This imagination exercise can be done over and over and in different areas of your life. If you center an imagination exercise on your career, first start with that first day at college or university, trade school or work experience. Be sure to take the complete journey, through your dorm room, friends, class, clubs, weekends, evenings and mornings. At the end of the journey, you might just find yourself wanting a different career path. Always focus on the inspiration, joy and love that you are experiencing to understand if you are on the correct path.

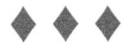

BELIEVING IS SEEING

(Inspiration, love, joy)

Earlier in our journey we not only learned about your 'Oh Yea! That's me!' Moment, Desire, Want or Need, you should have taken the time to discover it, write it down and read it, repeating it multiple times a day and when needed every hour.

As you stay vigilant to this habit you will find yourself daydreaming about the Joy you are finding on your way to Happiness. Every day that you continue the habit of writing down or saying out loud your 'Oh Yea! That's me!' moment you will see yourself not only enjoying your journey but experience the milestones of joy, smiling, laughing not only to yourself, but with friends, family and acquaintances.

The more you can see yourself in the ideal situations you want and the more you join in and participate in the journey, then your beliefs will become realities. The key is first being able to know why and what you want. You may want to know if you can join in and participate in the journey before you know why you really want to, and the answer is yes. It is yes for this reason alone; you may not think you know why, however just the fact that you decided to join the journey holds the simplest reason that you know you have the capability to be happier and want that for yourself.

What most people find along the journey is that their dreams get bigger and they start reaching and discovering more reasons they want to be happy. Let's take a few minutes to write down our 'Oh Yea! That's me!' Moments, Desire, Wants and Needs.

PILLAR #3: PLEASURE

Pleasure - Something to Think About
(gratitude, contentment, satisfaction)

Pleasure - Tough Stuff
(gratitude, inspiration, hope, interest,
awe, serenity)

Pleasure - Just for Fun
(amusement, interest, fun, joy, delight,
gladness, glee, enjoyment, happy)

Pleasure is often the only aspect associated with being 'Happy'. The easiest of the Pleasure family is found under 'Just for Fun' and supplies you with the immediate feelings of joy, smiles and laughter. Most people think this is the complete definition of happiness.

This however is only surface happiness and often leaves you as quickly as the moments in which we experience the gift, joke, funny situation, pet video. This is why Pleasure is the last ingredient because it is the toppings to happiness, not the foundation to creating a truly 'Happy' life. Even though it is the last ingredient, there are three fundamental areas of pleasure; Something to Think About, Just for Fun and the Tough Stuff. The easiest, as you may have guessed is 'Just for Fun' and is often how many describe and try to obtain 'Happiness', however this one single area is fleeting moments of happiness and is not sustainable for creating a happy life. One cannot spend their entire day watching videos of cats, dogs, babies and special people tricks! These can be superb in creating a smile, but we do need to explore and understand the other two areas of Pleasure as well as laying the foundation with the first two pillars of a 'Meaningful Life' and 'Your Purpose'.

Let's begin the first area of Pleasure – Something to Think About.

PLEASURE – SOMETHING TO THINK ABOUT – IS IT LIFE OR DEATH

(gratitude, contentment, satisfaction)

Is It Life or Death?

When was a time you were sparked with anger or cursed under your breath? How about an over-powering anxiety or frustration moment? Would it be nice if you didn't have these minor setbacks? What about the thought, "I don't need one more thing to happen!".

Believe me, in those moments the pain or anxiety is real, but can it just as easily be put away? The answer is yes, but it does take quite a bit of work.

Can you make a quick list in your head of these situations and in each of these instances, ask yourself the question?

Is this life or death?

What percentage of these situations would the answer be "Yes", it is life or death?

Now, by all means if it is a life and death instance and you are still alive, it is time to be completely and totally filled with gratitude and absolutely no self-pity.

In all those cases that the answer is "NO" ……. it isn't life and death, you will have to work at changing your reaction, it is time to brush it off and learn to treat each of these situations with gratitude that it is not life threatening, so not really worth your time to worry, be upset with yourself or the other person.

In one of the upcoming chapters, you will learn how to stop playing the Rerun. Stop the Rerun is great to use once you decide this is not a life or death situation.

When you find yourself in one of these very tense moments, try to quickly stop the hurt, anger, anxiety, frustration by coming up with a single word that you can say or think at that very moment. The funnier the word, the better this works. If it takes repeating your word 3, 5 or 10 times until the calm settles in, that is perfect. Over time you will find yourself only needing to say the word once. As more and more time passes and you practice this and many of the happiness habits, you will very seldom, if at all, find yourself having these stressful moments because truly, not much that we encounter on a daily basis is 'life or death'.

PLEASURE – THINK ABOUT – CAN IT BE WORSE?

(gratitude, contentment, satisfaction)

Can It Be Worse?

All throughout our lives we are faced with many small, medium and really big tragedies. What is the best way to handle these hitchhikers on the journey to Happiness?

As these hitchhikers appear on your journey take a minute and ask yourself this question. Can this be worse? Unless it is a life and death situation, it usually can be worse. This is not to belittle the challenge you have or are experiencing, but to help you put the situation into perspective.

If what has happened to you involves death, I send you my sincerest sympathies and this is truly not a hitchhiker situation. Take the time to go through the grieving process and work through some of the simpler happiness tasks.

However, if it could truly be worse, then thank your lucky stars, hug yourself and keep going. Say out loud that you are so thankful and that it could be worse will be better than just thinking it.

In the beginning you may find yourself repeatedly asking 'Can this be worse?' so many times per day that it may feel like you are getting nothing done other than answering this question. Do not let this discourage you, instead let it be an encouragement that you have decided to become a much more positive person, and this is a path that will help you learn to live your best life. You may not realize how negative you have become, however once you start asking yourself this, it may become quite clear. The good news is that you can and will eventually turn your thought process around.

Instead of being anxious or frustrated you will begin to take on an attitude of gratitude, knowing that you are quite lucky as most any situation could be worse, and you find contentment in knowing this. It does take practice and time to get to this stage, keep practicing even if you have setbacks.

The power of this question may not only bring you to a happier place, it may also inspire you to reach out to help others that are worse off.

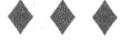

PLEASURE – THNK ABOUT – UNWIND AND BE KIND

(gratitude, contentment, satisfaction)

Unwind and Be Kind

As you move through this journey to Happiness, there will be some days that you move fast, days that you will move slow and other days you will skip altogether. While taking on the tasks in this book, you are meant to work them into your life so that they become habits. Some will be done hourly, others daily or weekly and the goal would be for the 'bad' habits to disappear altogether.

Rest assured that the happiest people still have a few days or seasons that they have to work on their journey also. What this means for you is that you will find that occasionally you will get rusty in these habits and need to work on them again.

When was the last time you did a kind act? Has it been today? Yesterday? Last week?

There are many kind acts that can be done every day or at least once a week. This simple thought of finding the time to be kind may very well overwhelm you. Please don't take it that way. Some of the simplest kind acts can be sending a text to say hi to a friend or acquaintance. If you can carve out the time to pick up the phone and say Hi that is even better because of the connection in real time with a person. Better yet, plan on meeting a friend out for a real conversation, movie, adventure or shopping trip.

From there you can move up to bigger and bigger kind acts. Read below to get some ideas and feel free to come up with your own.

- Compliment someone
- Open doors, even if you have to slow down and wait for the person to get there
- Hold the elevator
- Write a note, however small
- Pick up trash you see laying around
- Buy someone breakfast
- Hail a taxi for someone
- Let someone know if they have a tag sticking out
- Smile at someone you pass by
- Collect soda can tabs for charity or cereal box labels
- Volunteer through a group
- Volunteer to help your neighbor
- Read to a child
- Read to an elderly person
- Spend time with someone
- Run a much-needed errand for someone
- Make a gift basket
- Hand make an item
- Write Thank you notes
- Write letters to people in senior care facilities
- Say 'I love you'

PLEASURE – THE TOUGH STUFF

(gratitude, inspiration, hope, interest, awe, serenity)

This will be the toughest section of the book because it holds information you may not want to read or hear. It reviews the hard things in life, the truly tough stuff. It is much easier to fall into the everyday grind and feel sorry for ourselves, live in our own drama or that of the world around us.

Some of the toughest situations in life is learning to control the experiences we can and to let go of the ones' we cannot control. These next few sections will help in trying to handle the tough stuff so that your feelings of gratitude, inspiration, hope, interest, awe and serenity grow beyond all you have imagined.

PLEASURE – TOUGH STUFF – GRATITUDE SWAP FOR SELF–PITY

(gratitude, inspiration, hope, interest, awe, serenity)

Gratitude Swap for Self-Pity

We have all fallen into the age-old trap of self-pity, those moments when we either believe what others are saying or what we tell ourselves about a situation we are in or bad moments we are experiencing.

Why is it we fall into self-pity? Do we want others to feel sorry for us? Does it give us an excuse? Does it allow us to give ourselves an excuse? Does it give us a reason for doing some undesirable behavior? For all of these questions the answer can be yes and it is often for each of the situations we find ourselves basking in self-pity.

There is absolutely no reason for self-pity, no matter what happens. As long as you are alive and breathing then you have the opportunity to change your circumstance. Yes, it may be difficult. Yes, it may take so much energy, time and endurance that you question if it is worth it.

You have a choice every time you begin to feel self-pity; you can look for the positive and be grateful it isn't worse, you can change your situation, or you can wallow in self-pity. Happiness has no room for self-pity.

In order to stop self-pity in it's track, you must always be on the lookout to end this useless emotion before it starts. Next it is best to have a few tools ready until self-pity no longer invades your days. One of the tools to use against self-pity is to ask yourself – Could this be worse? Get over the self-pity and be grateful that it wasn't worse. Another great tool is to list all the people that are worse off than you. Get over your self-pity and go help someone worse off than you. Make small, medium and big goals for your life. Now when self-pity creeps in, pull out your goals and begin or continue to work on any of them. Another great tool to attack self-pity is to go through all the positives in your life.

There are so many people out in this world that are lacking in one or more ways that never feel sorry for themselves and the thoughts of feeling sorry for themselves doesn't cross their minds. On the other hand, you will find people who are decently well-off moaning, whining, groaning and complaining about their lives.

At any point that you feel self-pity creeping into your thoughts or life, stop and take however long it takes to go through all the things you have to be grateful for today. Even if you don't think you can come up with one, remember you woke up this morning and two, you have the ability to change anything. Next, reflect on the first 2 pillars of Happiness, purpose and meaning, and if you haven't already begun building or finished those pillars, now would be the time to start. You should now be able to swap your self-pity with mountains of gratitude.

The first few times you are faced with swapping self-pity with gratitude it may be difficult or over-whelming, remember it is ok to just take it a small step at a time to conquer this useless emotion. When you get rid of self-pity you will be forever grateful.

PLEASURE – TOUGH STUFF – SET GOALS

(gratitude, inspiration, hope, interest, awe, serenity)

The Description of you –Set goals

Setting goals for yourself is great! One of the main reasons why is because you are always in control. Want to change your goal? No problem, it is a goal of yours so change it. Your goals are one of the things that you have complete control over. There will be a challenge though if you try to change someone else's goal or if you let someone change your goals.

Feeling overwhelmed? If so, then start out by just setting small goals followed by the actions it takes to achieve those goals. No one says you must spend long, boring hours trying to determine your entire life goals. Start with something small, something you can accomplish this afternoon or this week. If for any reason it does not work out the first time, set a new goal and try again. Your commitment to yourself and your goals must be strong, even if you falter, pick yourself back up and renew your commitment daily.

By reading or listening to this book, whether you realize it or not you have picked a goal to 'Improve Your Happiness'. You can take the chapters that apply to you and they can become your actionable items once you supply a timeframe for accomplishment to the tasks contain in each.

Remember goal setting is just the first step, you must assign actionable items to your goals to ensure that your goals are met. Once you begin to accomplish the small goals your hope and interest will grow due to the sense of accomplishment and pride that will blossom through each goal.

So exactly how do you go about setting goals? First, decide what your priorities are in your life. Not everything can be a priority, or nothing will get done. Listed here are the most popular priorities that you may want to consider setting goals for:

- Spiritual
- Intimacy
- Family
- Home
- Physical Health
- Emotional Health
- Financial
- Work or Career
- Education
- Community
- Fun
- Social Life
- Environment

Pick 1 or 2 priority areas to set 1 or 2 goals that motivate you, are actionable, measurable, attainable and that can be accomplished in a stated timeframe. The most important thing is that the goal must motivate you. If it doesn't, you really will not accomplish your goal. If you look outside yourself for approval and sense of achievement, it will be hard to find deep satisfaction in your achievements.

After you have set your goals, you must define tasks that will help you achieve your goals. Tasks are not all created equal. Some tasks will give you quick wins, while others will spring you forward, and others need to be done first because of their importance or other tasks are reliant on them.

Once you have defined your goals and tasks, write them down, keep them in view and not tucked away in a document in the cloud, on your phone or computer or desk drawer. Make them your background screen, put them on your calendar or simply tape them up where you can see them every day.

PLEASURE – TOUGH STUFF – GIVING UP CONTROL

(gratitude, inspiration, hope, interest, awe, serenity)

If You Can't Control It – Forget About It

The irony of control and constantly trying to control our lives or others' lives thinking it will make us happier, sabotages our happiness instead. Once you let 'control' get a strong hold on you, you may find yourself trapped.

Having some control in our lives is natural and good. It is when we take too much control that we lose control. You know you have lost control because you begin to attach yourself to outcomes you planned, instead of what shows up as the most valuable or productive outcome. Having a plan is great and often necessary, we must also learn to stay flexible, open and letting go of some of the control so that you can experience more joy, peace, happiness, connection and freedom.

Why do most people feel they have to control more than they should? FEAR.

Fear is the number one emotion behind control and taking control too far, which then erupts many other negative emotions; Anger, Sadness, Shame, Jealousy, Disgust.

TRAP: you feel too much FEAR, in order to feel less fearful and more in control, you begin slowly but surely trying to control everything around you. The downward spiral begins, and you become the most incredibly efficient, getting things done with incredible ability and micromanaging until you are completely stressed out.

Learning to handle and manage control is possible with the right tools and habits.

Understanding what causes us to feel the need to control others, situations, circumstances, money, details, hold on too tight and other important parts of our lives. Fear, feelings of unworthiness, and lack of trust are the foundation of control. The stronger these feelings results in a deeper foundation in which control is housed. Learning the process to not be as controlling or give up some control is simple but may not be truly easy. You may not know how to let go or what it looks like, however, you have to be a willing participant and want to be willing to let go of some of the control.

Contain your fears by adjusting your expectations. Often fear is based on the worry that things won't turn out, that bad things will happen, or we will be hurt if we don't try to control people, situations, environment or circumstances. What are your expectations you have for yourself? What are the expectations you have of other people or the world? Your standards may be so high that neither you, nor anyone else can meet them. It is time to bring them down to a reasonable level. Often you need a friend or family member to speak with and figure out what is reasonable. Remember, getting to an expectation is a journey and you are looking for progress and not perfection. Be patient with yourself or others. Focus on what is improving, not what is going wrong or falling short of your expectations.

Contain your fears by imagining the worst-case scenario. Address the elephant in the room by thinking and writing out the worse-case scenario. Once you write out the worse-case scenario, it often is not that bad and something you can handle, and it is not a major catastrophe.

In order to begin giving up control we must be willing to count on others, to believe that things will be okay without us micro-managing every aspect. If you control everything, there is little chance that you can accomplish everything you are trying to control, let alone take on anything else. Even if things aren't done exactly like you would do them, it will be done good enough in many instances. By allowing someone else to take on a few tasks, even if it isn't how you would do things, you will be less stressed and anxious. Decide ahead of time if the task is important for you to handle or not. If it isn't absolutely necessary for you to handle, ask someone else to do it. Be ready to be surprised, that even though someone may not perform a task exactly like you would or at the speed you would, they may exceed your expectations or at least save you the time of doing it yourself. Remember, when you let someone help, don't micromanage, give them a chance to do it their way, thank them for their efforts and avoid criticizing them.

Trust yourself to begin trusting others. Embrace gratitude for others and for yourself. Remind yourself that you can handle this and that letting go is hard, but it's worth it. Remember letting go of control will be hard and you will think staying in control is so much easier. Get yourself out of the spiral, live through the harder times of letting go until it becomes a habit.

PLEASURE – TOUGH STUFF – NO DRAMA

(gratitude, inspiration, hope, interest, awe, serenity)

Kick Out the Drama

Do you have drama in your life? Do you really want to be drama free?

Why do we create or wallow in drama? It provides a comfort zone, a place to blame everyone or everything but ourselves for our problems. We are attracted to drama when we are bored and have too much free time in our lives. Also, when we have too much negativity in our lives we are drawn to and more susceptible to drama. Getting rid of the drama is not an easy task, it takes good habits to break the drama habits and become happy and drama-free.

Until you decide to be drama-free, you may not even realize that you are in a drama filled world. You could be living in other people's drama or be the one that is creating the majority of the drama. Drama has become a norm as most reality TV shows promote real-life drama and make you feel like you are missing out if you don't have your own drama days. Drama can be enticing because you may feel it energizes you, however this will eventually turn into fear, sadness and anger. Deciding to give up drama could be one of the biggest decisions you make as you may feel like you are missing out. Remember, drama kills your creativity and playfulness, two things that make life much more fun and happier.

So exactly how do you give up drama? Changing your habits and becoming aware will be the biggest allies to kick drama out of your life.

If you are complaining, moaning or groaning; then you are probably contributing to your own or someone else's drama. Practice catching yourself and immediately change the subject to a more positive conversation. This is tougher than it seems, so take the time to come up with subject changers ahead of time. The best subject changers are those in which you compliment someone or ask them what the best place, restaurant, movie that they've seen in the past month. Having this list of subject changers memorized also helps when someone else is the complainer, moaner or groaner. As quickly as possible, interrupt nicely and ask them one of the subject changer questions. You can also be ready with a quick joke or funny, pleasant or adventuresome story of your own.

There is no time for gossip, not listening to gossipy stories and no repeating the gossip. The old saying applies here, 'If you don't have anything good to say, don't say anything!". So, what do you do when someone starts in with a gossip story? There are several things you can do; change the subject, simply speak up and say you don't participate in gossip or interrupt with a compliment about the person in the gossip story. This will usually stop the gossiper right in their tracks because you have indicated you really like the person that the gossip was going to be about. Whatever you do, do NOT give in to listening to the story because that would mean you gave in to the drama. Make a firm commitment to avoiding drama at all costs and distance yourself from people who have or create too much drama.

One of the reasons we seem to find ourselves in a drama filled situation is because we have taken things personally. Understand that most people act the way they act because of who they are, not due to something you did or said. Realizing that someone's words or actions have more to do with them than you, you won't feel the need to engage in their drama. The next time you feel like you are being judged or attacked, step back, breath deep and do nothing or walk away and remember that you do not have to react to their actions or words.

Another way to look at a situation where someone has said something or appeared to be mean or ugly to you is to give them the benefit of the doubt. Maybe they just received terrible news about a friend or family member or even themselves. We all wish we could deal with negative news better, but it just isn't possible for many. Don't automatically assuming that being cut off, rolling of the eyes or being snapped at was caused just by something you did, said or looked, giving someone the benefit of the doubt will ease the situation and diffuse most drama.

We mean well when one of our friends is confiding in us and we begin to give them our helpful unsolicited advice. This is one of the surest ways to begin drama and is one of the challenges with posting and social media. We post something on a social media site that we are passionate about and suddenly, we have haters telling us how our opinion is all wrong. Think about it, was there a question in the post asking for advice or opinion? Most of the time there isn't, yet there will be many posts that stir drama and arguments. It is actually good to see our friends' points of view so that when we meet out it is much easier to engage in pleasant conversations and steer clear of those subjects that our opinion is different.

Letting people know casually that you don't 'do' drama and keeping the high road by positive conversations or not speaking ill of anyone or repeating unfavorable information will often keep you out of the drama zone. Keep focus on what you want and knowing that you are in charge of your own feelings will help you with the habits to remove drama from your life.

PLEASURE – TOUGH STUFF – NO TIME FOR RERUNS

(gratitude, inspiration, hope, interest, awe, serenity)

Don't Binge Watch Your Past

Isn't it easy now to binge watch movies, TV series repeatedly? Do we all have that DVR in our heads? You know the one that pops up and replays a piece of our past in which we wish we would had done something different. How many times have you replayed that same video? Let me give you the cold, hard truth ..... just like a movie, TV episode or even a video you took with your phone; your past story is not going to change, no matter how many times you replay it, it is the past.

This is one of the hardest habits to break, to forcibly catch yourself beginning to play the old memory that makes you cry, that has you saying 'If only', 'Wish I would have', or that makes you feel like you want to punch someone. You will have to come up with a trigger to interrupt the memory and all the what-ifs you put yourself through. Your trigger will have to be something that can be done anywhere as these memory reruns are relentless at popping up at any and all times until you make the habit to stop them.

My trigger was to say the word "STOP" out-loud and replace the rerun memory with plans that I was going to do that night, that week or my next vacation. There was a point that I stapled post-it notes with the word "STOP" to the handle of my purse to remind me. It helped me break the habit faster because do you know how silly it looks to have post-it notes stapled to the handle of your purse?

In the beginning the rerun will get most of the way through and you will start playing the what-if game – STOP the rerun. Over time you will be able to catch the rerun at the beginning. Over time you will never have reruns and only be looking toward the future and great memories to be made. You may think that this is impossible, however, trust me it isn't. Once they go away, a small miracle occurs because they rarely come back.

If you noticed this is a task that takes quite a bit of time and effort, however, it is really important to do this for yourself. The good news is, you are in total control, not reliant on anyone or any place. The hard news is, you are in total control. If you have a close friend that you can call when a rerun begins and they know the goal to stop the rerun and help you change the subject, have a good laugh or chat about anything else, this may also be a solution for you.

PLEASURE – TOUGH STUFF – JOURNAL TIME

(amusement, interest, fun, joy, delight, gladness, glee, enjoyment, happy)

Time to Write or Just Act

I know you may have heard this a hundred times before, yet you may learn one thing that you didn't know about the benefits of keeping journals. This falls under tough stuff because it takes time and it is truly just about you. Why this is challenging is because when it comes to making ourselves a priority, we often do not give ourselves the time and energy we need.

Journaling can be beneficial in as little as 15 minutes 3-5 times; this is confirmed in the study *Emotional and physical health benefits of expressive writing.* Expressive writing is just free-flow writing with no worries on punctuation, spelling, and grammar. On that same idea, a separate *study by the University of Iowa* goes on to say that the benefits are better when expressed in a story form.

In addition to an expressive journal that may be filled with the good times, anxious times, bad times, funny times and all the other times in your life, think about starting a second journal called 'Me and My Awesomeness'. In this journal make sure you write something, even if it is only a single word daily.

The third journal to have is a Gratitude Journal. To journal gratitude or not to journal gratitude is left up to you. Personally, I like to action my gratitude most of the time and keep a partial gratitude journal. To action gratitude can be anything from sending appreciative texts, to coffee, a sticky note or a full–blown email or thank you letter. The ideas are endless if you are more of a doer versus a writer. So why do I keep a partial journal? Some days I just don't have time, or at least don't think I have the time and it is easier to just be grateful that I woke up, found my glasses or remembered to take the trash to the road on the correct morning.

Some of you may be wondering why a gratitude journal. In this day and age of being surrounded by the negative news and world events, bombarded by news on the television, phone, and computer we may feel terribly unhappy and ungrateful. Instead of running to the latest gadget, fad diet or your next big thing, try writing in your Gratitude Journal. Starting a gratitude journal is easy because there are already so many good ones online if you want to begin using something already laid out. If you have your own journal whether it is online or on paper, you can always use 'gratitude prompts' if you are having issues coming up with gratitude ideas. Whether you list 1 or 3 things you are grateful for every day, start today, even if it is on a scrap piece of paper. An attitude to take on, though it may be one of the hardest things you do, is to know that you are owed nothing and should be grateful for everything.

PLEASURE – JUST FOR FUN – PLAY

(amusement, interest, fun, joy, delight, gladness, glee, enjoyment, happy)

I am about to surprise you with a fact. Most people believe that these feelings; amusement, interest, fun, joy, delight, gladness, glee, enjoyment, and happy are the only thing that makes up happiness. Unfortunately, though these feelings are an important part of being happy, you cannot sustain lifelong happiness with only this piece of pleasure. You must have the first 2 pillars, Meaning and Purpose/Why, and the other 2 parts of the third pillar pleasure, and the feelings that go with them.

Maybe you already know how exhausting it is to be in constant search for and trying to experience the feelings for this part of pleasure thinking that this is the only part of happiness? Perhaps you have been dissatisfied with your partner because they can't keep up with trying to keep you in these feelings? Knowing that this is simply the 'play' part of being happy and not necessary for everyday should bring you peace. Now that you have read about the first two pillars, Meaning and Purpose/Why, and the first two parts of pleasure, you know that true happiness takes effort, wisdom and habits.

The good news is that this is one of the easiest parts of pleasure and being happy. The funny part is most of us need reminders that we can be an adult and still play which brings about most of these feelings.

Play and fun can be done in big and small ways. The first thing you must do is relax and make sure you have practiced your smiling and laughing, huge parts of these feelings. Play also varies dependent upon our individual personalities, likes and dislikes and play personality, as researched by Dr. Stuart Brown. Depending on your personality, you may find that you need additional groups of friends and acquaintances in order to find your fit for this area of pleasure. Have you ever found yourself in an activity that everyone else is enjoying but you? It could just be that this activity didn't fit your play personality.

Dr. Stuart Brown theorizes that there are 8 play personality types. We have all met the Joker or class clown in our lives, or maybe that is you. Next is the kinesthete, like the athlete, though not competitive, that involves the need to keep moving. The explorer loves new experiences whether it is physical, mental, emotional or relational. The competitor's goal is to win or being the best. As a director loves organizing and dictating the flow of work and play. The collector collects, it really is that simple. The maker of things is the artist/creator and the final type is the storyteller.

Knowing which play personality you fall into will help you understand what truly brings you pleasure when it comes to play and possibly work, more about that later. You may find yourself falling into 1-3 categories or just a single category. There is no right or wrong category that you fit into for play. Remember also that just because an activity does not fall into your specific play personality, you can still have fun and enjoy yourself. This will also answer your doubts when you find yourself having absolutely no fun while everyone else is having a wonderful time.

Playing can be big or small, free or expensive or somewhere in-between. It may sound simple, but having a list of ideas, spouse, friends with the same play personality, Meetup groups or Facebook friends will help you fulfill this area of pleasure and some or all the feelings that go with it. If you and your spouse, children or close friends are different play personalities, you can now help them with their play personalities and activities that will bring them the play pleasure feelings. Remember, just because something doesn't specifically fit into your play personality, you might find great pleasure from it and may be just what your friend needs. Have fun, smile and laugh as playing will bring you much happiness.

Listed below are more details about the play personalities:

Joker – Class clown, funny person, funny jokes and stories

Kinesthete – on the move, inside or outside, long or short walks, runs, bikes, swims or many other activities.

Explorer – adventures big and small, in real life or researching

Competitor – compete in all different ways, online games, in person physical, mental or relational

Director – organizer big and small, master of tasks

Collector – keeps collections of things or resources, research

Artist/Creator – doodler, writer, singer, musician, depends on art medium

Storyteller – writes, tells, listens to stories, podcasts, blogs, vlogs, movies

When it comes to play, it can be planned or spontaneous, some of the fun times are not planned, last minute and free.

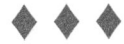

PLEASURE – JUST FOR FUN – HAPPY MOMENTS

(amusement, interest, fun, joy, delight, gladness, glee, enjoyment, happy)

This area of pleasure is just those moments that bring a happy thought, smile, squeal of joy, quiet and big belly laughter. For everyone these moments can be so different for each of us. These are perhaps the moments that you lived for before thinking that they were all there was to happiness. Wanting someone else to cause the smile on your face, the glimmer in your eyes or the music to your ears on a constant basis to keep you in a good mood.

Don't get me wrong, these moments are truly meant to be cherished, looked forward to and relived throughout our lives. What you will have learned by now is that you can bring these moments to yourself whenever you need them. These moments will build on the foundation you have set by understanding and working on your Happiness Pillars #1 and #2, Meaning and Purpose/Why.

At this point, you will have learned that you do not need to exhaust yourself trying to create happy moments for the family and friends in your life on a constant basis. If you are around someone that looks to you to 'make them happy', you will know that you are not responsible for the happiness. You can and should of course include them in your fun times so that they can experience some sun, some of your third part of pleasure. You will also have a resource you can share with them so that can begin to understand true happiness and how to achieve it. You, of course, can become the most fantastic role model.

BONUS MATERIAL:
HAPPINESS HABITS

How to Grow Your Happiness

LIVE working on making a best life for you

LOVE that you learn to stop comparing

HAPPY that growing up doesn't mean growing old

xoxoxo

HAPPINESS HABIT #1

Smile at Someone

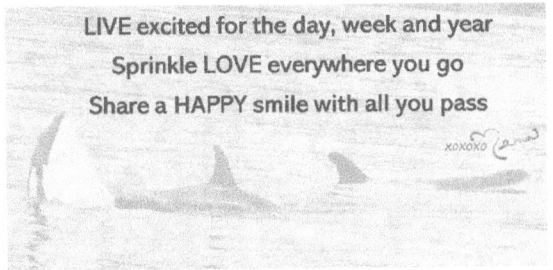

Sometimes we must catch ourselves to see if we are in such a hurry that we scurry through life, not looking up, not looking at anyone and not taking in the scenery or the people around us.

If you already look around while you are out, waiting to catch another's eye to find just the right moment to give them a smile then this chapter is an easy skip for you.

However, if you have gotten out of the habit of looking up as you go to your work desk or area this will be a great time to try a game of catching someone's attention and just simply smiling and nodding your head. If you don't have the opportunity or are not in the situation to catch someone's attention going to or leaving work, then there are a couple of other opportunities to practice the smile exercise.

The next time you are at the grocery store take the time to go up and down the aisles or stop in front of the bakery display case. I am sure there will be someone that will be available to smile at whether you are checking out all the different types of apples you can buy now or looking at all the new and different kinds of cereal that are taking up all the shelves in the grocery store. Follow the delicious scent of homemade bread and bakery items all the while looking for the opportunity to smile at one of the wonderful bakers making these delightful items.

As you simply make small connections by the simple small nod of your head and smile on your face you will find a smile being returned, a conversation started, or even the starting of a new wonderful friendship.

HAPPINESS HABIT #2

Making 'How Are You Count'

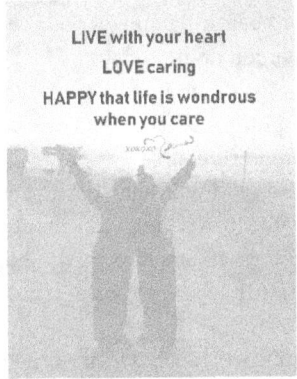

LIVE with your heart

LOVE caring

HAPPY that life is wondrous
when you care

Some days for some people talking to people is just asking too much. When you are ready and perhaps even before you are ready, you must challenge yourself to go beyond the smiling and nodding at complete strangers.

Even though my friends and acquaintances would swear I am an extrovert, I am not really. Over time due to owning my own businesses and needing to make sales, I have found a wonderful trick that allows me to have interesting encounters with others and fits my introvert style.

There are three things to do; two to say and the most important one left is simply listening. Not just hearing, but active listening. You may not have heard of active listening, so I will do my best to ensure you know exactly what I mean before you finish this chapter.

Since active listening is much, much harder than the two things you have to learn to say, we will start with the two things to say.

First thing to say, 'How Are You?'

The first thing to practice is simply ask someone how they are. Now I have learned to do this so that it prompts for positive answers, as being in the positive is so much easier to work with on the journey to Happiness.

Examples of how to ask someone how are you?
- What is the best thing that's happened today so far?
- What would be the best thing that could happen to you today?
- What was the very best thing about this past year?
- What would make this day be wonderful for you?
- How are you and that beautiful smile of yours doing?
- How is my favorite person doing today?

Now if you are at the beginning of your journey you may feel or think this is really just too corny. Be patient with yourself as you will soon understand that if you just ask a person how they are, you will hear mostly negative comments. Now, we don't have time for that on our journey and we actually not only want to be on the happiness journey ourselves, but we are also in the business of helping others on their happiness journey whether they know it or not.

Second thing to say, Compliments ...... and they are Free.

Compliments are one of the easiest things to give that is free, however not many of us choose to give something that costs us nothing.

But wait, it does cost you. It costs you time, time that it takes to look around, stop and notice your surroundings, look around, notice your surroundings, catch someone's eye, smile and pick up something about them, what they are wearing, driving, saying, looking at one of their features and then talking to them by giving them a compliment.
Now here comes the remainder of the opportunity to giving someone a compliment.

To actively watch their expression and actively listen to what they say after the compliment.

I realize this takes the most valuable commodity we have, our time. This simple fact that it takes our precious time is why compliments have become a rare gift. With our busy life and so many responsibilities we often don't feel we have the spare time. Believe me, if you make the time to give a compliment beginning once or twice a week, you will soon realize how much it is doing you good on your happiness journey. Think about this, what if you were given a compliment 1-3 times a day, let alone a week?

A compliment brings smiles, goodwill, conversations, laughter and friendships. A compliment strengthens character of the giver, goodwill towards each other and that warm feeling on the heart of the giver and receiver.

Now for the HARD Part

So, you've creatively, positively asked "How are You?" And you have given them a compliment. What comes next is the hardest part for almost everyone. Clear your mind, look the person in the eye, small smile and actually listen to what they say. Truly listen, no interrupting, no thinking about what you want to say next, actually listen and ask them a question about what they just said or make a statement concerning anything positive that they just said......or simply give them another compliment.

HAPPINESS HABIT #3

Do a Favor

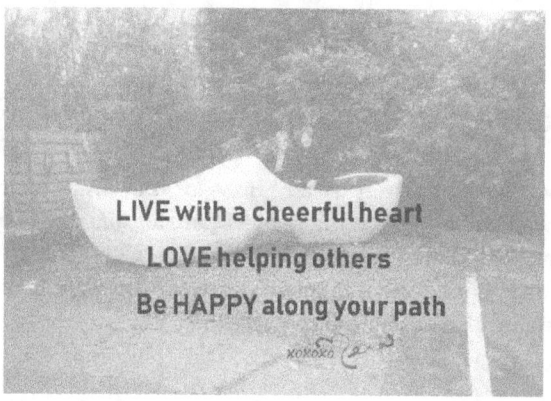

LIVE with a cheerful heart
LOVE helping others
Be HAPPY along your path

Have you ever found yourself with too little time and too much to do? Would you believe that other people also find themselves in this same predicament? Or have you ever found yourself not quite having the expertise to do something that to someone else is quite easy? Would you believe that you have talents that other people cannot do and perhaps could use some help?

This is one of those habits that is simple but may not be too easy for several reasons. One, you may not have actually considered giving your time to your neighbor, church, family or friends. Two, you may think you just don't have any time to give. Or three, you may not think there is anything that you can do for anyone.

One way to get into the habit of doing favors is to actually ask someone for help or a favor, whether it is an actual task or just their opinion. Reaching out to others is a great way to let them know you are open and willing to reciprocate and help them when possible.

Try it today, you may just find yourself smiling, laughing and enjoying the outcome.

HAPPINESS HABIT #4

Be the Inspiration to Someone's Journey

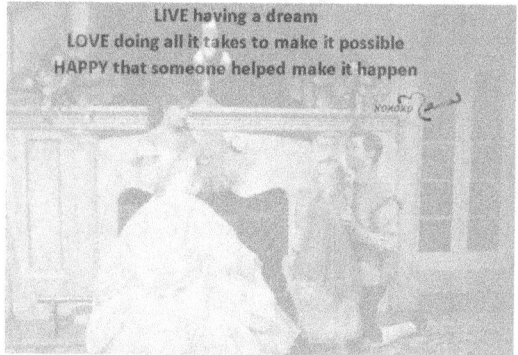

Often, we do not realize the number of people we impact daily. Sometimes just doing our job to the best of our ability is a true inspiration and motivation to others. It could be just having a wonderful, positive conversation with someone and actively listening to them as they share a piece of their past with us is an inspiration for them to move forward on their happiness journey. There are many times that others may hear us that we don't even know they are listening, that we become an inspiration for them.

Make sure you tuck the negative away, learn the 3 pillars of happiness and become a role model that other people want to emulate. Care about your impact on this world, country, city, neighborhood, home, family and friends. The way you live your life will soon become someone's greatest inspiration.

HAPPINESS HABIT #5

Put a Little Light in Your Day

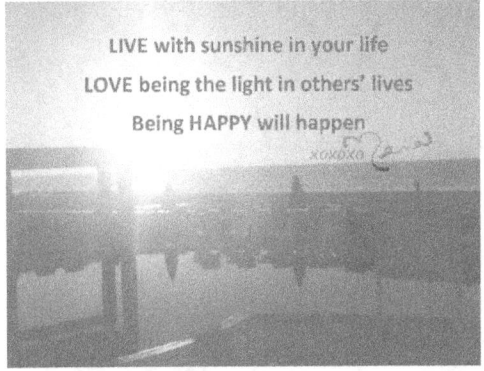

In this fast-paced world, desk jobs and binge-watching TV series, there is little time spent outdoors. And then there is the time change and how that can throw your whole life into a frenzy. Part of the year you may be going to work in the dark and part of the year you don't get home until dark.

A little bit of sunshine goes along way if you can and will just take the time to get outside, look up to the sky and smile, even if it is only 10 minutes a day or every other day. And, remember even if it is overcast, the sun is always shining above the clouds and you will still reap the benefits from going outside.

Plants are not the only things that need and grow in the sunlight.

Benefits of 5 – 15 minutes of Sunlight a day:
- Natural serotonin boost – want more happiness, boost your serotonin.

- Natural sunlight gives us Vitamin D which is heart healthy, can lower cholesterol and blood pressure and may help to prevent the onset of diabetes.
- Kick away the Winter's blues (SAD – Seasonal Affective Disorder)
- Warms your body's muscles which can ease stiffness and reducing pain caused by inflammatory conditions
- Boosts your immune system

THANK YOU AND ENJOY YOUR JOURNEY

True Happiness

LIVE today beginning your journey
LOVE all the steps, easy and difficult
Know that being Happy is a worthy goal

xoxoxo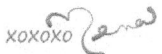

www.ingramcontent.com/pod-product-compliance
Lightning Source LLC
Chambersburg PA
CBHW062158290526
45791CB00016B/1004